Sweet Dreams

Sweet Dreams
A Guide to Productive Sleep

Frank Minirth, M.D.
Paul Meier, M.D.
Richard Flournoy, Ph.D.
Jane Mack

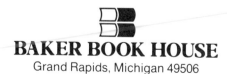

BAKER BOOK HOUSE
Grand Rapids, Michigan 49506

Contents

Introduction

Sleep is an interesting phenomenon, to say the least. In general, it has been poorly understood through the years. A few people have claimed they needed very little sleep. Many people have probably been criticized for sleeping too much. A lack of sleep has been said to represent a "troubled mind." Others maintain that their lack of sleep represents, not a "troubled mind," but a "troubled body." In recent years, with the discovery of brain waves, researchers have understood more and more about many aspects of sleep, especially dreams. Indeed, in recent years more and more is being written on both a scientific and popular level about factors affecting sleep. In this booklet some of those factors are summarized with our suggestions for improving sleep. We have tried to give practical tips. The booklet is especially written for the Christian. Christians may, as anyone else, have problems with sleep. However, the problems can be overcome. We hope the following information will prove helpful.

1

Statement of the Problem

Can you help me? I can't sleep," a distinguished Christian leader said as we began our discussion. She was suffering from one of America's leading problems: sleeplessness.

There are currently over seventy million people in America suffering from sleep disorders. An estimated thirty million have severe sleep disorders. An extremely conservative estimate is that at least 20 percent of Americans suffer from an extended period of insomnia during their lives. Christians, as well as non-Christians, have this problem. We see literally thousands of individuals in our counseling clinic each year who suffer from sleeplessness.

No doubt a person with insomnia has felt like Job when he stated:

> When I lie down I say,
> "When shall I arise?"
> But the night continues,

And I am continually tossing until
dawn.

(Job 7:4, NASB)

2

What Is Sleep?

There is a rhythm and harmony, a balance and equilibrium, in all our bodily functions and in all we think and do. Sleep is one of these important cycles. Very little is actually known about the nature or physiology of sleep, but it is unquestionably an inherent function of the body or we would not be spending one-third of our lives in this state.

There is a special area in the brain, in the hypothalamus, that has been provided to supervise our sleep. Therefore, we know that sleep is an absolute necessity. Other areas of the brain that probably also play a part in our sleep and wakefulness cycle are the reticular activating system, the ventral portion of the frontal lobe, the midlobe thalamus, the hypocampus, the amygdala, the lower brain stem, and the pineal gland (Groves and Schlesinger, 1979). Also, the neurotransmitters serotonin, acetylcholine, norepinephrine, and dopamine play a role.

Sleep could be defined as a state of mind

when the body is at rest, and there is a natural suspension of consciousness. The brain is constantly emitting electrical waves, and the nature of these electrical waves actually changes during sleep. In fact, there are four different levels of sleep, each emitting different brain waves; and there is even a more interesting brain wave emitted when a person is dreaming.

In summary, sleep comes when both the body and the mind are to some degree at rest. As stated above, there are interesting electrical changes in the brain during this period.

3

Why Is Sleep Important?

One-third of our lives is spent in sleep. If one goes without sleep for several consecutive days, personality changes, irritability, and depression can take place and even psychosis can develop. During World War II, when the enemy wanted further information from our captured troops they would repeatedly awaken our men as soon as they would go to sleep. After awhile, the men would have severe mental problems and would confess almost anything. Sleep deprivation proved a tormenting punishment (*American Handbook*, 1974). Also, experiments in which animals were deprived of sleep for a length of time resulted in the animals' deaths (Carlson, 1981).

The brain works incessantly during a person's waking hours, and it is provided with a rhythmic timing mechanism which requires it to suspend operations to some degree after approximately sixteen hours of continuous activity. One theory is that the brain simply needs time to recuperate its vital powers (Carlson, 1981). Just resting in bed will not accomplish this. A sound sleep is required for the higher centers of the brain to get perfect rest. As long as we are awake, the brain is not at rest, no matter how much our muscles are resting. Another theory states that we need sleep to metabolize certain chemicals that are built up during the day (Carlson, 1981). In other words, sleep is also physiologic and biochemical. In either case, sleep is a necessity.

Regular hours of sleep are essential to health and renewed energy for the next day. The vast majority of people need seven to eight hours of sleep per night. Most individuals who claim they can get by on less are simply using denial. Thomas Edison was a famous individual who probably fit in this category (Kepler, 1980). He was a firm believer in little sleep. However, he failed to emphasize the fact that he made up for sleeping less at night with frequent naps during the day.

Efficiency and effectiveness decrease with sleep loss. For example, during World War II, Great Britain increased the work week to help meet the demands of war. The idea worked until the week was extended beyond fifty-four hours. Beyond this limit, and with resulting overwork and sleep loss, production actually began to decrease (Kepler, 1980).

The individual who can get by on six hours of sleep or less per night is an extremely rare exception to the rule. In fact, the individual who gets less than four or five hours of sleep per night has a sevenfold increase in the chance of dying at any point in time.

Another interesting observation made by researchers is that individuals who tend to sleep too much are likely to be "worriers" (*Comprehensive Textbook*, 1980). They worry over everything.

4

Causes of Insomnia

Insomnia is the inability to fall asleep. One who suffers from insomnia cannot fall into a restful, deep sleep or wakes up after a short sleep and then lies awake the rest of the night. Researchers have found that those who regularly lose sleep over a period of time may require many weeks to recuperate and regain their former mental and muscular efficiency and precision (Carlson, 1981). Extended wakefulness causes a dulling of the mind and a depression of all the body functions. Insufficient sleep often results in a loss of appetite, indigestion, constipation, anemia, loss of weight, and can be followed by a lowered resistance to infections and diseases. Regular as well as sufficient sleep is absolutely necessary for effective work and good health.

Anxiety and Stress

Like all rhythmic functions of the body, the rhythm of regular and sound sleep can be upset when a person is worried or tense. Anxiety and stress are underlying causes of over 95 percent of all cases of insomnia. Insomnia in turn increases the stress. Overcoming insomnia can aid in overcoming stress.

Anxiety, the chief cause of insomnia, could be defined as an emotion characterized by fear, apprehension, and dread. The anxious individual is in emotional turmoil and feels something must be done. The anxiety may be accompanied by such symptoms as tremor, irritability, rapid heart beat, sweating, being hyperalert, nervous stomach, sighing respiration, or hyperventilation (*DSM III*, 1980). The individual is worried and can't concentrate.

Anxiety usually, but not always, accompanies depression. Depression, in contrast, is characterized by a sad expression and behavior accompanied by painful thinking.

Depression

The second cause of insomnia is depression. Whereas insomnia is often reflected by difficulty in falling asleep, depression is often reflected in early morning awakening. The depressed individual often has no motivation, low energy, and feels blue.

Anxiety and malocclusion are the chief causes of bruxism (teeth grinding through the night). About 20 percent of people grind their teeth at night (*The Dallas Morning News*, April 30, 1984). For this problem the anxiety should be dealt with in counseling, and a dentist should also be consulted. Good results are often obtained.

Age

In general, as age increases, the need for sleep decreases to some degree. Older individuals can be expected to sleep less than when they were young. Actually, many older people do not need much less sleep; they just sleep more lightly (Kepler, 1980). They are awakened more easily. They may have more pain (arthritis, neuritis) and not sleep soundly. They often make up for less sleep at night by napping during the day. A newborn baby sleeps most of the time (approximately 18-20 hours per day, with 50 percent of that time spent dreaming). Babies will gradually sleep less and less as they grow older, finally stabilizing in the teen and adult years. As stated before, the majority of adults need seven to eight hours of sleep per night. However, some individuals feel very refreshed on less sleep than this. Again, a word of caution should be given to the individual to be sure that six hours of sleep a night is really sufficient. Some denial might be present.

Stimulants

Caffeine, which is contained in many beverages (coffee, tea, sodas, chocolate), is a stimulant. Consumption of more than 600 mg. a day can cause insomnia in many individuals. Excessive caffeine taken near bedtime is often a problem. Ulcer medication, high-blood pressure medication, and birth-control pills are other substances that may keep individuals awake.

Exercise near bedtime will cause an adrenalin release, having a stimulating effect and causing insomnia. Also cigarettes contain nicotine (a stimulant) and can cause insomnia. Amphetamines ("uppers") are street drugs used to help a person "stay awake." They are stimulants and can seriously disrupt normal sleep for many days.

Habits and Personality

Many individuals cannot sleep because they are afraid that they cannot sleep. Fear of not sleeping becomes a habit. It actually produces a conditioned response which keeps the individual awake. When psychiatrists and psychologists tell these same people to try to stay awake for several hours each night on purpose, a psychological phenomenon known as "paradoxical intention" occurs, especially in perfectionistic individuals. Most of them will fall rapidly to sleep in spite of their previous history of insomnia and in spite of their new efforts to stay awake. The minds of perfectionists (who are frequently the oldest child of their sex in their families) are constantly involved in obedience-defiance conflicts, as described in our book, *The Workaholic and His Family* (Minirth, et al., 1981).

Perfectionistic individuals are compulsive, hard-driven, "type A" personalities

(Minirth and Meier, 1978). They have trouble turning off their minds. But all personality types *can* have trouble sleeping.

Sleeping Position

Some individuals sleep in an awkward position that actually causes insomnia. They may sleep with one leg under the other or an arm bent under their head. The position may need to be changed. Sleeping on a firm support mattress helps people sleep better.

Noises and Light

Some individuals have trouble sleeping because of noises. We do not get used to noises as many believe (Kepler, 1980). The bedroom needs to be quiet and with as little light as tolerable. Some children and adults feel safer with a small nightlight; and this is, of course, no problem.

General Physical Problems and Pain

Many individuals have chronic physical problems and pain which, of course, makes sleep difficult. Headaches (caused by anxiety, certain foods, allergies, physical disease) keep many people awake. Other diseases that may be associated with sleep difficulties include thyroid disease, seizures, hypoglycemia, and cerebrovascular disease. More rare causes include pickwickian syndrome, Kleine-Levin syndrome, or brain tumor (Tomb, 1981).

Specific Physical Problems

Sleep apnea is a medical disorder which can be caused from a central problem in the brain itself, shutting off respiration; or it can be caused by a peripheral obstruction of the respiratory tract, which is seen in some individuals who snore (*Comprehensive Textbook,* 1980; Tomb, 1981; Kepler, 1980; Orr, Roffway, and Williams, 1981). Some of these individuals with the peripheral obstruction may benefit from surgery of the respiratory tract. Also, some individuals with sleep apnea benefit from a medication known as Vivactil. A doctor should be consulted. Sleep apnea has been blamed for "crib death."

Nocturnal myoclonus (involuntary jerking of legs) keeps some individuals awake (Kepler, 1980; Tomb, 1981). About 20 percent of insomniacs suffer from this jerking. Medication will help some cases.

Another mysterious condition known commonly as "restless legs" will keep some people awake at night (Kepler, 1980; Tomb, 1981). The legs may tingle, itch, and want to move. A doctor should be consulted for this as for other medical problems that keep individuals awake.

Another very interesting condition known as *narcolepsy* will cause some individuals (one out of every 2,000) to have poor sleep at night (Tomb, 1981; *Handbook of Clinical Behavioral Therapy*, 1981). This condition is characterized by: daytime sleep attack, catalepsy, hypnagogic hallucinations, and sleep paralysis. The daytime sleep attacks are brief (few minutes) but can be dangerous since they occur during activity. The catalepsy is a loss of muscle tone that is usually precipitated by strong emotions. The hypnagogic hallucinations usually occur as the patient is falling or going to sleep. They may be frightening. The sleep paralysis occurs as the patient is falling asleep or awakening. He or she is fully conscious but can't move. Medications can often help in narcolepsy.

A fifth category that can result in some individuals having poor sleep is nightmares or night terrors (*Handbook of Clin-*

ical Behavioral Therapy, 1981). With nightmares there are frightening dreams with vivid recall (REM or dream sleep). With night terrors there is intense anxiety and vocalization but no recall since it occurs during stage IV sleep. Psychotherapy may be indicated and medication often helps.

Finally, other specific problems that affect sleep include *jactatio capitis nocturna* (head banging), somniloquism (sleep talking), bruxism (teeth grinding), somnambulism (sleepwalking), and enuresis (bedwetting) (*Handbook of Clinical Behavioral Therapy,* 1981). Behavior modification techniques and medication can help in enuresis. A medical doctor or psychiatrist may need to be consulted in head banging, sleep talking, or sleepwalking. A dentist can be of help in bruxism.

Irregular Patterns

A source of sleeping difficulty for some people is irregular times of going to bed and getting up the next morning. Going to bed at different hours may contribute to insomnia, because the body gets used to (or tries to get used to) sleep at a certain time. Also, persons with deep disturbance would be better off sleeping according to their natural biological rhythm (early to bed or later to bed) instead of retiring early if they are a "night owl." Natural biological rhythms (circadian rhythms) do vary from individual to individual (Groves and Kurt, 1979).

5

How to Get Restful Sleep

1. Exercise

It seems that exercise early in the day probably has both psychological and chemical effects that do help individuals sleep. Exercise should not be done late at night, because with exercise one gets an adrenalin release; which could actually prevent sleep.

2. Stimulants

Caffeine and cigarettes can also be stimulants and can keep one awake. These should be avoided especially late at night.

3. L-tryptophane

This is a precursor of serotonin, a brain chemical that controls sleep. Research has shown that L-tryptophane has apparently been of benefit to some people. This amino acid has been called "nature's sleeping pill" and can be found in dairy products, fish, poultry, and meats. It can also be purchased at drug or health food stores, but to date has not been FDA approved. Consult a local physician regarding the value of using this for a particular individual.

4. Warm milk and honey just before bedtime

This old technique drawn from grand-mother's recipes actually does have merit (Kepler, 1980). Blood is drawn to the stomach and a sleepy sensation is created by the decreased blood flow to the brain. Warm milk really can help.

5. Hot bath and massage

These will help to decrease tension, which will aid in muscle relaxation and help induce sleep.

6. No work in the bedroom

Many hard-driving individuals have paperwork or other business materials in the bedroom. This produces a conditioning response of anxiety, and sleep inhibition can occur just by entering the bedroom. The bedroom should be used only for relaxation, marital pleasures, and sleep. One should look forward to going to bed without feeling the strain of work.

7. Techniques

Certain techniques are helpful in slowing down a rapid-thinking mind (*The Dallas Morning News,* April 1984; Turner, Calhoun and Adams, 1981). For example, one might picture himself or herself with a giant piece of chalk writing on a huge blackboard, starting at one hundred and counting down toward one (counting sheep really does help). Some persons imagine being all wrapped up in string or rope and relax their muscles one area at a time as they imagine the string unwinding from that area of their body. Others imagine God's hand being larger than their bed, then imagine themselves lying peacefully in God's hand, meditating on John 10:27–31, which reassures us that believers are eternally secure in the hands of Christ and God the Father.

8. Physical cures

Physical causes such as sleep apnea need to be ruled out. Many people snore because air passages are shut off when they lie horizontally. This may be severe enough to actually awaken a person several times during the night. Surgery may be helpful in such cases. A medication called Vivactil may help when snoring is a problem. A doctor should be consulted.

A doctor may also be of assistance in

dealing with other physical causes of poor sleep: narcolepsy, nightmares, night terrors, bedwetting, head banging, sleepwalking, bruxism, nocturnal myoclonus, restless legs, thyroid disease, seizures, hypoglycemia, and cerebrovascular disease.

9. Relaxation exercises

Listen to relaxation tapes, one per day for three months combined with the repeated message, "Anxiety is a signal to relax," to condition the brain to relax and fall asleep. Alternately tense and then relax every muscle or muscle group in the body starting at the head and working down to the feet (or vice versa, depending on your preference). Breathe deeply and then relax while exhaling and counting down from 10 to 0. Tell yourself with each number down, "I am going deeper and deeper to sleep."

Another relaxation technique that can

be of tremendous aid to sleep is a varia-
tion of Benson's original relaxation response that consists of the following: Lie
quietly in bed with your eyes closed, lights
out, and all other necessary bedtime rit-
uals completed. Then let all of the muscles in your body relax deeply from the
tip of your toes to the top of your head.
Take three s-l-o-w, d-e-e-p breaths, breathing slowly and deeply through your nose,
gradually becoming more and more aware
of your breathing. Every time you exhale,
silently say to yourself one of the
following:

> sleep
> rest
> peace
> calm

or any other one-syllable word. Continue
breathing easily and naturally at your own
pace for ten to twenty minutes or until
you drift off into normal, natural sleep.

Practice this every night at bedtime, and in a matter of a few days you should find yourself falling asleep much more quickly, easily, and restfully. Many people continue practicing this relaxation procedure indefinitely or every night for the rest of their lives as part of a healthier, calmer bedtime ritual.

10. Avoid drugs

Many sleeping medications disturb stage IV sleep, which is a very important part of sleep. Thus, more sleep probably becomes less productive. Also nearly all effective sleeping medications produce tolerance (requiring more and more) and withdrawal symptoms on cessation of medication. Thus after one month these medications (minor tranquilizers, sedatives, barbiturates) are utterly worthless. They have often been used effectively for short periods in times of crisis, and their use should be limited to such circumstances. Sleeping pills can make drug addicts out of normal people.

Rather than using sleeping pills obtained through a prescription, some individuals buy over-the-counter sleeping pills. These pills often contain an antihistamine, which is sedating. However, they can have negative side effects (even psychosis) and are not without drawbacks. Those containing bromides are especially dangerous.

11. Avoid alcohol

Many people use alcohol to go to sleep. In fact, literally thousands do. Alcohol is America's number-one abused drug. The alcoholic beverage industry now enjoys sales of fifteen billion dollars annually. The individual who uses alcohol to induce sleep should be aware of the potential abuse factor and that alcohol reacts dangerously with many other drugs. Daily alcohol usage actually lowers the brain's serotonin level, causing increasing sadness, decreased sex drive, and insomnia. Insomnia that results from this type of depletion is usually in the following pattern: The individual falls asleep relatively easily but wakes up a few hours later and requires one or two hours to fall back asleep. This will occur every other night or more often in individuals who have low serotonin levels.

12. Don't worry about it

Although loss of sleep is extremely frustrating, no one ever died from loss of sleep. One of the biggest factors that keeps people awake is worrying about being awake. Don't worry about relaxing or sleeping. Let yourself maintain a passive orientation and permit yourself to relax and sleep. Don't try to make it happen. Allow relaxation, rest, and sleep to occur at a natural pace. If distracting thoughts occur, ignore them and repeat *rest, sleep,* or *calm* over and over to yourself as you breathe out. If after awhile you can't sleep, then get up, leave your bedroom and read the Bible or a relaxing book until you feel sleepy. Repeat this process if necessary and until sleep occurs within fifteen to twenty minutes.

13. The bedroom should be well-ventilated

Have an ample supply of fresh air during all seasons (*The Dallas Morning News,* April 1984). But it is important that strong drafts be avoided. For most people, a temperature of 64 to 69 degrees Fahrenheit aids sleep. If it is too warm, most people will sleep less and toss more.

14. Don't hesitate to see a Christian psychiatrist or psychologist for therapy

Research shows that the major psychiatric problem that keeps people awake at night is depression. This sleep disturbance is characterized not only by difficulty in falling asleep, but also by early morning awakening. In fact, if only difficulty falling asleep exists, the problem is probably anxiety related. Research shows that these depressed individuals tend to internalize their emotions with resulting sleep problems. They can thus benefit by insight-oriented psychotherapy as well as anti-depressive medications, most of which are not at all addicting or habit-forming.

Anxiety results in depletion of brain amines (serotonin and norepinephrine) with resulting sleep problems. This imbalance can be corrected in two or three weeks with antidepressant medications which are not addicting and produce no tolerance or withdrawal. A person either has a chemical imbalance or does not. If a person does have a serotonin imbalance, it can be simply corrected. A side effect of the antidepressant medication is that it is also sleep producing. If given at bedtime, it will serve as a good sleeping pill. However, the antidepressant medications should *never* be used unless the person taking them is also receiving psychotherapy.

The primary cause of over 90 percent of insomnia and 90 percent of depressions is repressed anger or repressed guilt (anger at self). The individual is frequently not even aware of the repressed anger or guilt, but it is easily uncovered by a professional counselor with experience and good techniques. Repressed anger is the primary cause of serotonin depletion, and serotonin depletion is the biochemical cause of 90 percent of insomnias and clinical depressions. Seeing a well-trained

Christian psychologist will result in uncovering the repressed anger or guilt, dealing with it biblically (ventilating, forgiving), and learning how to avoid ever developing insomnia or depression again. (Study the book, *Happiness Is a Choice*, for more details on this.)

Over half of all Americans will go through an insomnia-producing, clinical depression sometime in their lives. About 10 percent of Americans require a psychiatric hospital stay of one or two months sometime in their journey through life in order to overcome a serious clinical depression. The odd thing is that wonderful, hard-working, overly-conscientious people are the most prone to insomnia and depression. That is probably because they are the most likely not ever to admit to themselves that they are feeling angry when they have daily disappointments.

Ephesians 4:26 tells us that anger is a normal emotion and that we can become angry without sinning but must forgive by bedtime. Antidepressant medications can speed up the serotonin re-uptake and thus get the depressed individual with insomnia back to work and back to a happy life sooner. But if therapy is avoided, the root problem (subconscious anger or guilt) will cause insomnia and depression to keep coming back when the antidepressant is stopped. The root problem must be resolved.

15. Avoid eating a heavy meal right before retiring

This can cause physical discomfort and keep one awake. Also, drinking a "night-cap" will backfire on some people and actually result in fitful sleep.

16. Noises

Just as most noises keep individuals awake at night, a few noises make certain individuals sleep very well. For example, many individuals can benefit by the sound of a fan in the background.

17. Healthy rituals

Never just flop down and try to fall asleep. Instead, make it a rite and a pleasure. Do various personal tasks that will help you to terminate all contact with your daily affairs of business, work, and worries. Attend to your mouth hygiene, bathe or just wash your face, massage your scalp, etc. Some people try singing, humming, or whistling during this personal time. Going through the same activities night after night will condition or help one learn to fall asleep. For many married persons, sex has a relaxing effect before sleep.

It takes most people thirty minutes or less to fall asleep. However, some people are such "doers" that they can't stop reviewing the day's activities. The above sleep ritual might help such a person. It helps to train them to leave daytime pressures at the bedroom door. One mother used to say that at night she would put all of her concerns in a bag and pick it up the next morning—not a bad idea.

Also, keeping regular hours can help. It is usually best to have a set time to go to bed and a set time to get up, making as few exceptions as possible so the body can set its biorhythms.

18. Wear light, loose sleeping garments

Avoid heavy coverings to permit easy access of air to your skin as well as to your lungs. Use just enough covering to keep your feet warm and your body comfortable, but not hot. The free access of air to the skin helps to remove some of the poisonous oxidation products. Oxidation and expulsion of carbon dioxide are usually greater during rest and sleep. The air coming in contact with the skin also stimulates respiration and lung action.

19. Aspirin

Yes and no. Thousands of individuals take two aspirin at night to help them sleep. Aspirin does not help sleep per se, but it does help relieve pain that keeps many people awake. Recent research shows that it may also help the cardiovascular system and prolong life expectancy slightly. However, aspirin also irritates the stomach lining and causes slight bleeding in the stomach. Your family doctor should help you make this decision.

20. Peaceful music

You may find that listening to a favorite piece of music that is soothing and relaxing may help induce sleep. Try listening to classical or other "easy listening" music at a lowered volume just prior to retiring for the evening. This can be a cue or part of your preparation for a good night's sleep.

Also, many a saint through the years has found sweet sleep from one of the old hymns of the faith. These are just a few old favorites.

Blessed assurance, Jesus is mine!
Oh, what a foretaste of glory divine!
Heir of salvation, purchase of God,
Born of his Spirit, washed in his
    blood.

This is my story, this is my song,
Praising my Savior all the day long;
This is my story, this is my song,
Praising my Savior all the day long.
                Fanny J. Crosby

What a friend we have in Jesus,
    All our sins and griefs to bear!

What a privilege to carry
   Everything to God in prayer!
O what peace we often forfeit,
   O what needless pain we bear,
All because we do not carry
   Everything to God in prayer!
                Joseph Scriven

Nearer, still nearer,
Close to thy heart,
   Draw me, my Savior,
So precious thou art.
Fold me, O fold me
Close to thy breast;
   Shelter me safe
In that haven of rest.
              Mrs. C. H. Morris

God moves in a mysterious way
   His wonders to perform;
He plants his footsteps in the sea
   And rides upon the storm.

Ye fearful saints, fresh courage take;
   The clouds ye so much dread

Are big with mercy and shall break
   In blessings on your head.
             William Cowper, 1772

He leadeth me: O blessed thought!
   O words with heavenly comfort
   fraught!
Whate'er I do, where'er I be,
   Still 'tis God's hand that leadeth
   me.

He leadeth me, he leadeth me;
   By his own hand he leadeth me.
His faithful follower I would be,
   For by his hand he leadeth me.
           Joseph H. Gilmore, 1862

Sun of my soul, thou Savior dear,
   It is not night if thou be near;
O may no earthborn cloud arise
   To hide thee from thy servant's eyes!

When the soft dews of kindly sleep
   My weary eyelids gently steep,
Be my last thought, how sweet to rest
   Forever on my Savior's breast!

Forgive me, Lord, for thy dear Son,
  The ill that I this day have done,
That with the world, myself, and thee,
  I, ere I sleep, at peace may be

O may my soul on thee repose
  And with sweet sleep my eyelids
    close,
Sleep that may me more vigorous
    make
  To serve my God when I awake.
              John Keble
             Bishop Ken

21. Watch Naps

We have noted that some individuals who enter the hospital suffering from insomnia are napping a lot during the day. When they eliminate those daytime naps, they sleep much better at night.

22. Interpreting your dreams

It would be foolish to put too much importance in your dreams. Some people have had a bad dream, falsely assumed that it was God leading them, and then made major, foolish, life-altering decisions based on that bad dream. People are the authors, producers, and directors of their own dreams. We dream about things that we are concerned about on an unconscious level. God can and does teach us insightful things through our dreams sometimes, but our decisions should be based on something more dependable, like God's Word and the advice of wise counselors.

Our dreams can be about things we are afraid of, but usually they are exaggerated wish fulfillments. If I have a dream in which I am killed or harmed in some way then, when I wake up, I assume that I am probably feeling somewhat guilty on a deep inner level. Punishing myself in that dream satisfies my guilt feelings. Therefore, I pray for insight so I can figure out what I am feeling guilty about, then deal with that guilt biblically. If someone else is hurt or killed in my dream, then I assume that I probably have some repressed anger toward someone (usually of the same sex as the imaginary person in my dream). I pray again that God will reveal to me who I might have repressed anger toward, then I forgive that person, whether or not they deserve it for the Lord's sake. I may also confront that person if it would be beneficial.

Case Study

One of our patients was suicidally depressed but had no idea what he was depressed about. He was asked to write down his dreams that week. He had a repeated dream in which he hitchhiked. A married couple picked him up in a car with no outer body, the car hit a bump, the husband fell out, and my patient drove off with the other man's wife. Then he got out of the car himself and was chased by his father, who was trying to punish him. The patient was shocked when he was told that his suicidal depression was probably caused by repressed guilt over an affair with a married woman. He said that was correct; he had had a brief affair six months earlier. He prayed for God's forgiveness.

23. Meditation on the Psalms and other Scripture

Just before and when one initially lies down, the mind can be very easily influenced. Whatever is read or seen at that point can have a powerful influence on the brain and subsequent behavior. The influence can range from violence on television to a soothing psalm, which reflects security. Which is better? Below are eleven scripture passages (NASB) out of hundreds that have brought comfort to many people over the years as they have wrestled with sleeplessness.

There is therefore now no condemnation for those who are in Christ Jesus (Rom. 8:1).

And we know that God causes all things to work together for good to those who love God, to those who are called according to *His* purpose (Rom. 8:28).

In this is love, not that we loved God, but that He loved us and sent His Son *to be* the propitiation for our sins. Beloved, if God so loved us, we also ought to love one another. No one has beheld God at any time; if we love one another, God abides in us, and His love is perfected in us. By this we know that we abide in Him and He in us, because He has given us of His

Spirit. And we have beheld and bear witness that the Father has sent the Son *to be* the Savior of the world. Whoever confesses that Jesus is the Son of God, God abides in him, and he in God. And we have come to know and have believed the love which God has for us. God is love, and the one who abides in love abides in God, and God abides in him (1 John 4:10–16).

Who shall separate us from the love of Christ? Shall tribulation, or distress, or persecution, or famine, or nakedness, or peril, or sword? (Rom. 8:35).

Finally, brethren, whatever is true, whatever is honorable, whatever is right, whatever is pure, whatever is lovely, whatever is of good repute, if there is any excellence and if anything worthy of praise, let your mind dwell on these things (Phil. 4:8).

In peace I will both lie down and sleep, For Thou alone, O Lord, dost make me to dwell in safety (Ps. 4:8).

God is our refuge and strength, A very present help in trouble. Therefore we will not fear . . . The Lord of hosts is with us (Ps. 46:1,7).

Peace I leave with you; My peace I give to you; not as the world gives, do I give to you. Let not your heart be troubled, nor let it be fearful (John 14:27).

Be anxious for nothing, but in everything by prayer and supplication with thanksgiving let your requests be made known to God. And the peace of God, which surpasses all comprehension, shall guard your hearts and your minds in Christ Jesus (Phil. 4:6–7).

Therefore do not be anxious for tomorrow; for tomorrow will care for itself. *Each* day has enough trouble of its own (Matt. 6:34).

The Lord by wisdom founded the earth; By understanding He established the heavens. By His knowledge the deeps were broken up, And the skies drip with dew. My son, let them not depart from your sight; Keep sound wisdom and discretion, So they will be life to your soul, And adornment to your neck. Then you will walk in your way securely, And your foot will not stumble. . . . When you lie down, your sleep will be sweet (Prov. 3:19–24).

6
Summary

We will all spend a third of our lives here on this earth sleeping. And yet very few individuals take the time or effort to be sure this big portion of their life is developed productively. How well we take care of the sleeping third determines how productive we will be during the two-thirds of our lives that we are awake.

God created sleep and created the need in humans for sleeping and dreaming. Psychiatrists and psychologists use dreams as "windows" to see what is going on in the unconscious dynamics of their patients. They also use sleep patterns to help determine root problems (repressed anger, and so on) that need to be uncovered and resolved. Trouble falling asleep, for example, usually means the person has emotions or motives he is afraid to face. Looking at these hidden emotions and motives in therapy, then dealing with them biblically, results in decreased anxiety and improved sleep.

On the other hand, if an individual falls

asleep relatively easily, wakes up fairly often at 3:00 A.M., and can't get back to sleep for one or two hours, the experienced psychologist knows immediately that the individual *probably* has a serotonin deficiency in his or her brain, caused by the root problem of holding in some repressed anger or guilt. By verbally probing the person, together they can uncover the root problem, deal with it biblically, and the serotonin problem will straighten itself out naturally when the root problem is truly resolved. If the symptoms are severe and the individual feels like he or she can't cope with work or family pressures, then the Ph.D., psychologist, will refer that individual to an M.D., psychiatrist, for antidepressant medications and/or a month or so of intensive daily therapy on a hospital psychiatric ward for total recovery from the depression. The psychiatrist will then refer the individual back to the psychologist for outpatient follow-up to be sure the old patterns of dealing with emotions are not reestablished.

For some individuals, insomnia is a simpler problem that can be resolved by making some of the other modifications outlined in this book and maintaining a balanced life physically, emotionally, and spiritually. Many of the scientific discoveries on serotonin have been made in the past decade. The authors of this brief, self-help book hope that our fellow Christians everywhere will integrate true scientific findings with biblical principles to better their enjoyment of life as well as the productivity of their lives, both while awake and while asleep.

References

American Handbook of Psychiatry 1974. Edited by Silvano Arieti, vol. 1, New York: Basic Books.

Carlson, Neil R. 1981. *Physiology of Behavior*. Boston: Allyn and Bacon.

Comprehensive Textbook of Psychiatry 1980. Edited by Jarold I. Kaplan; Alfred M. Freedman; and Benjamin J. Sadock, vol. 1, Baltimore and London: Williams and Wilkens.

Groves, Philip, and Schlesinger, Kurt 1979. *Biological Psychology*. Dubuque, Iowa: Wm. C. Brown Co.

Handbook of Clinical Behavioral Therapy 1981. Edited by Samuel M. Turner; Karen S. Calhoun; and Henry E. Adams. New York: Wiky-Interscience Publication.

Kepler, James 1980. *How to Get a Good Night's Sleep*. Chicago, Ill.: Bullong Press Co.

Minirth, Frank B. and Meier, Paul D. 1978. *Happiness Is a Choice*. Grand Rapids, Mich.: Baker Book House.

Minirth, Frank; Meier, Paul; Wichern, Frank; Brewer, Bill; and Skipper, States 1981. *The Workaholic and His Family*. Grand Rapids, Mich.: Baker Book House.

Orr, William C.; Roffway, Howard P.; and Williams, Robert L. May 25, 1981. Sleep Disorders. *Audio-Digest Psychiatry*, vol. 10, No. 10.

Quick Reference to the Diagnostic Criteria from DSM III 1980. The American Psychiatric Association.

The A to Z Guide to More Than 250 Different Therapies in Use Today 1980. Edited by Richie Herink. New York: New American Library.

The Dallas Morning News April 30, 1984. A Guide for Insomniacs: Getting a Good Night's Sleep.

The Harvard Guide to Modern Psychiatry 1978. Edited by Armand M. Nicholi, Jr. Massachusetts: The Balknap Press of Harvard University Press.

Tomb, David A. 1981. *Psychiatry for the House Officer.* Baltimore: Williams and Wilkens.